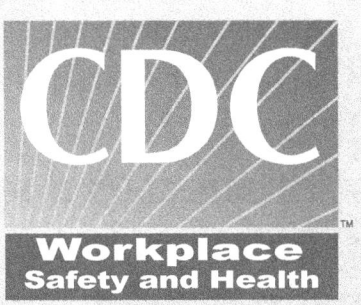

I0426384

Assessment of Mold and Indoor Environmental Quality in a Middle School – Texas

Nancy Clark Burton, PhD, MPH, CIH
John Gibbins, DVM, MPH

Health Hazard Evaluation Report
HETA 2008-0151-3134
July 2011

DEPARTMENT OF HEALTH AND HUMAN SERVICES
Centers for Disease Control and Prevention

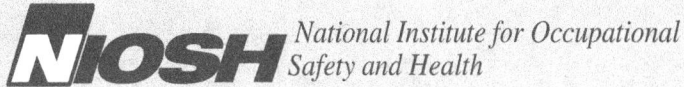

National Institute for Occupational Safety and Health

CONTENTS

ABBREVIATIONS

ACGIH®	American Conference of Governmental Industrial Hygienists
AIHA	American Industrial Hygiene Association
ANSI	American National Standards Institute
ASHRAE	American Society of Heating, Refrigerating, and Air-Conditioning Engineers
CDC	Centers for Disease Control and Prevention
CFM	Cubic feet per minute
CFR	Code of Federal Regulations
CO_2	Carbon dioxide
CO	Carbon monoxide
HHE	Health hazard evaluation
HVAC	Heating, ventilating, and air-conditioning
IEQ	Indoor environmental quality
IOM	Institute of Medicine
Ls^{-1}	Liters per second
NAICS	North American Industry Classification System
NIOSH	National Institute for Occupational Safety and Health
OEL	Occupational exposure limit
OSHA	Occupational Safety and Health Administration
PEL	Permissible exposure limit
ppm	Parts per million
RH	Relative humidity
U.S. EPA	United States Environmental Protection Agency
VOC	Volatile organic compound
WHO	World Health Organization

The National Institute for Occupational Safety and Health (NIOSH) received a management request for a health hazard evaluation at a middle school in Texas, which we had evaluated a year earlier. The request was to look at the indoor environmental quality (IEQ) at the school after mold remediation and remodeling had been completed.

What NIOSH Did

- We visited the school on April 22–24, 2008.
- We talked to employees about their health.
- We measured carbon dioxide (CO_2), carbon monoxide, temperature, and relative humidity (RH) in the school throughout the day on April 23, 2008.
- We collected sticky tape samples from surfaces to look for mold growth.
- We used thermal detection to look at temperature differences around window frames in the classrooms.
- We reviewed reports from previous environmental sampling.
- We talked about the results of an investigation done by the city health department that looked at student health issues.

What NIOSH Found

- The CO_2 levels in three classrooms were higher than recommended guidelines. This finding means there may be a problem with enough outdoor air being supplied to the classrooms.
- The air temperatures in the classrooms were lower than what is recommended as a comfortable level for indoor working environments.
- The RH levels in the classrooms were higher than what is recommended as a comfortable level for indoor working environments.
- The windows did not completely close at the time of our evaluation, so humid air could enter the building. All windows were replaced later in 2008.
- Small amounts of mold growth were found under wooden furniture and in the hallways.
- Complaints by staff about health symptoms have decreased following remodeling and mold remediation.

What Managers Can Do

- Provide at least the minimum recommended amount of outdoor air to the classrooms and library to reduce CO_2 levels. These recommendations are made by the American National Standards Institute and the American Society of Heating, Refrigerating, and Air-Conditioning Engineers.

- Follow current comfort guidelines for temperature and RH in the school. These guidelines are set by the American National Standards Institute and the American Society of Heating, Refrigerating, and Air-Conditioning Engineers.

- Inform employees and students about what is being done to address IEQ problems and why these changes are being made.

- Start an IEQ management program.

What Employees Can Do

- Get medical care for symptoms potentially related to your work. See a healthcare provider who is knowledgeable in occupational medicine and IEQ issues.

- Report any concerns you have about the work environment to management so they can address these issues.

SUMMARY

The school district had made many of the changes we and others had recommended. However, high humidity levels in the school remained and led to the recurrence of mold growth. We recommend that management modify the ventilation systems to ensure that IEQ parameters meet current guidelines and establish an IEQ management program.

In March 2008, NIOSH received an HHE request from management at a middle school in Texas concerning a history of mold contamination. NIOSH had conducted an HHE at this school in September 2007; the school was closed from September 2007 until March 2008 for repairs and mold remediation. NIOSH was asked to conduct a follow-up evaluation to look at the current IEQ conditions at the school.

In April 2008, we visited the school and looked at building conditions. We met with management and employees to discuss current issues. We measured CO_2, CO, temperature, and RH; used thermal imaging to look at temperature gradients; and collected sticky tape samples on furniture and ceiling surfaces to look for mold growth. At the request of the school district, the city health department conducted a parallel investigation to evaluate health concerns among the students.

We found that management had addressed many of the problems identified in the 2007 NIOSH evaluation including cleaning the ventilation units and repairing the annex flashing and leaking pipes in crawl spaces. The visible mold contamination had also been cleaned. However, we did find some areas of mold contamination on wooden furniture and in the hallways.

Air temperatures were below recommended ANSI/ASHRAE comfort guidelines, while RH levels were above ANSI/ASHRAE guidelines. Three classrooms had high CO_2 concentrations, which indicated that not enough outdoor air was being introduced into the space. Several of the windows did not close tightly, resulting in unconditioned air entering the school. Subsequent discussions with the school administration officials revealed that the windows in the school were replaced after our site visit.

When the school first reopened in March 2008, employees had headaches and nausea. These symptoms resolved after a short time and were thought to be related to the odors from the remodeling work. The employees reported that the classrooms were cold.

Some employees who had pre-existing allergies moved to other schools. The city health department found no differences in the frequency or type of visit to the school nurse for the students in the time frame of our evaluations.

Keywords: NAICS 611110 (Elementary and Secondary Schools), mold, allergies, relative humidity, carbon dioxide, temperature, indoor environmental quality, IEQ, ventilation

On March 18, 2008, NIOSH received an HHE request from school district management for a middle school in Texas. We had conducted an evaluation at this school in September 2007 (HHE 2007-0380) to look at IEQ issues including mold contamination and an incident involving employees inhaling chlorine while cleaning the ventilation system vents. The school district implemented many of the recommendations we made, and external consultants and asked us to conduct a follow-up evaluation at the school after it reopened in March 2008. We issued an interim letter in June 2008 with preliminary recommendations concerning the HVAC systems and windows.

Facility Description

The middle school opened in 1957 as a senior high school. The school campus consisted of five buildings: a two-story main building that housed the administrative offices, auditorium, band rooms, and classrooms; a two-story classroom annex; a physical education building containing the school swimming pool; and two additional buildings for maintenance and facilities. The main building and classroom annex (the buildings of concern) were built of concrete block and brick with interior plaster walls. The floors were poured concrete on grade or on a pier and post floor support system. There was a crawl space for utilities. Most classrooms had suspended fiberglass ceiling tiles. The hallways and stairwells had no mechanical ventilation and relied on pedestrian traffic for air movement. The main hallway of the main building had terrazzo flooring, and the rest of the flooring was vinyl or linoleum.

The administrative offices in the main building had a separate ducted ventilation system. The classrooms were served by individual unit ventilators mounted above the suspended ceiling. These units were installed in 2002. They were operated by a centralized system using thermostats in each of the classrooms. The ventilation units used a closed chilled or heated water system from the main utility building. Outdoor air intakes were located in external wall openings. The classrooms had functional windows, which were closed during our evaluation. The school had been closed from September 2007 until March 2008 for repairs and remediation. Prior to the school's reopening, the school district worked with an environmental consulting firm to ensure that the repairs and remediation had been completed.

ASSESSMENT

On April 22–24, 2008, we made a site visit that included an opening meeting with school district management representatives, representatives from the two unions representing teachers and staff, the school principal and assistant principal, school nursing staff, and representatives from the city health department. The city health department conducted a parallel investigation at the request of the school district to look at health issues among students.

Following the opening meeting, we walked through the main school building and the annex to look for evidence of water damage, water incursion, mold, and other potential IEQ problems. We collected data and reports from the school district management and seven sticky tape surface samples (SKC Inc., Eighty Four, Pennsylvania) on furniture and walls of hallways. The tape samples were sent to a commercial laboratory for mold confirmation and identification using direct microscopic techniques with lacto phenol cotton blue stain. We used Q-Trak™ Plus Indoor Air Quality Monitors, Model 8554 (TSI Incorporated, Shoreview, Minnesota) to measure CO_2, CO, temperature, and RH throughout the school day in five classrooms, the main office, and the library. The Q-Trak™ monitors were precalibrated and postcalibrated in our laboratory in Cincinnati, Ohio. A TRAMEX Moisture Encounter meter (Tramex Ltd., Littleton, Colorado) was used to qualitatively assess the interior wall moisture levels. A thermal imaging camera (Fluke FlexCam Ti55FT Thermal Imager, Fluke Corporation, Everett, Washington) was used to look at temperature differences in the exterior walls.

We interviewed 12 faculty and staff members who had been interviewed in 2007 to evaluate their current health concerns and occupational history. We also met with city health department staff to discuss their investigation of health symptoms and school nurse visits.

Building Survey

We found during the walk-though tour that some of the underlying moisture issues had been addressed. These included repairing the flashing at the back entrance of the annex to fix the ceiling leaks, installing a dual pipe system for the ventilation units, draining and sealing leaking pipes in the crawl spaces under the buildings, regrading the soil around the foundations, and completing the cleaning of the ventilation units. The visible mold contamination had been cleaned; however, some wooden furniture and cabinets and some surfaces in the unconditioned hallways looked like they had recurrent mold growth. We collected sticky tape samples in these locations (Table 1) and found active mold growth.

Table 1. Microscopic sticky tape sample results

Sample Location	Genera	Amount of Growth*
Room 113 – Bottom of wooden table	*Aspergillus/Penicillium* group *Aspergillus* spp. Hyaline hyphae	Many conidia/spores Moderate Moderate
Room 113 – Corner end table	*Aspergillus/Penicillium* group *Aspergillus* spp. Hyaline hyphae *Hyalodendron* spp. Ascocarps *Alternaria* spp.	Many conidia/spores Many Many Moderate hyaline conidia/spores Few Rare
Room 301 – Back of desk	*Aspergillus/Penicillium* group Hyaline hyphae *Aspergillus* spp. Ascopores	Moderate conidia/spores Moderate Few Rare
Hallway of Annex – Under ceiling tile	Hyaline hyphae *Aspergillus/Penicillium* group *Cladosporium* spp. Dematiaceous hypae	Few Rare conidia/spores Rare Rare
Room 306 – Door of cabinet	*Aspergillus/Penicillium* group *Aspergillus* spp. *Cladosporium* spp. Dematiaceous hypae Hyaline hyphae *Bipolaris/Dreschslera* group	Moderate conidia/spores Moderate Moderate Moderate Moderate Rare conidia/spores
Room 306 – Desk	*Cladosporium* spp. Dematiaceous hypae	Many conidia/spores Many

*Scale: many>moderate>few>rare

RESULTS
(CONTINUED)

We noticed that two ventilation units in the annex and one in the library were leaking water from the drainage traps; we reported them to the project manager who took steps to address the leaks. We also observed that the windows did not close tightly, and caulk was missing in several areas, allowing unconditioned humid outdoor air into the buildings. Figure 1 is a thermal image showing the leakage of warm air into the classroom. A gap was also visible between the edge of the window and the frame.

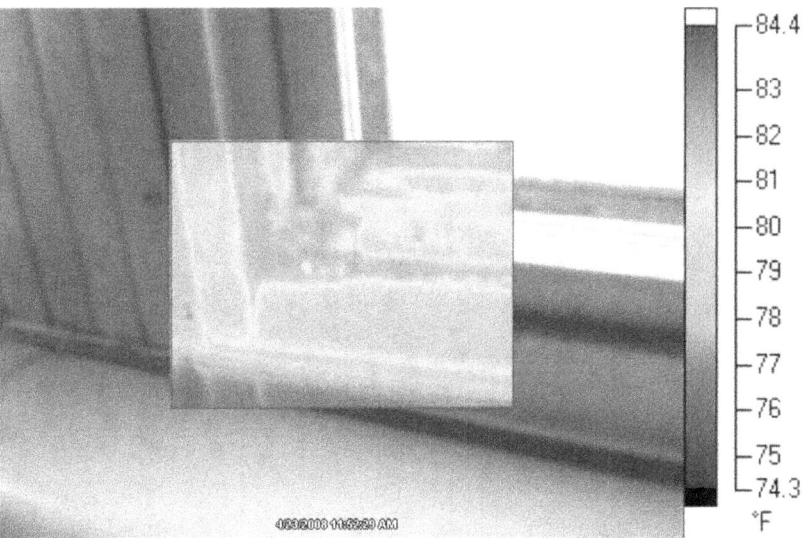

Figure 1. Thermal image of window in Room 305 shows outdoor air entering the room at a higher temperature than inside.

IEQ measurements (CO_2, CO, temperature, and RH) made during the site visit are summarized in Table 2. Graphs of the data for each room are in Appendix A. A spot check of outdoor conditions showed a CO_2 concentration of 405 ppm, a temperature of 87°F, and a RH level of 63%. Rooms 108, 203, and 212 had CO_2 levels above the recommended ANSI/ASHRAE guidelines [ANSI/ASHRAE 2010a]. CO_2, a normal constituent of exhaled breath, is not considered a building air pollutant. However, if CO_2 concentrations are elevated, the amount of outdoor air introduced into the ventilated space may need to be increased to dilute typical building contaminants. Rooms 111 and 213, which had the lowest CO_2 concentrations, were not occupied when the monitoring was done. The main office was on a central ventilation system and was operating within the ANSI/ASHRAE guidelines. CO levels were low, ranging from nondetected to 1.6 ppm. The presence of CO in the building may have come from vehicular traffic around the building. Additional information on IEQ including the ANSI/ASHRAE guidelines can be found in Appendix B.

RESULTS
(CONTINUED)

In Rooms 108, 111, 203, 212, 213, and the library, the temperatures and RH levels were outside comfort guidelines (Table 2). The ANSI/ASHRAE Standard 55-2010: Thermal Environmental Conditions for Human Occupancy, specifies conditions in which 80% or more of the occupants would be expected to find the environment thermally acceptable [ANSI/ASHRAE 2010b]. These guidelines have been established for comfort levels that can affect productivity, not on the basis of health effects. The current ANSI/ASHRAE guidelines also recommend maintaining RH at or below 65% [ANSI/ASHRAE 2010a]. Excessive humidity can promote the growth of microorganisms and dust mites. The moisture readings in Room 108, the teachers' lounge, and Room 410 showed no evidence of excess moisture on wall surfaces.

Table 2. Indoor environmental quality measurements made on April 23, 2008, at the middle school

Location	Sampling Time (minutes)	CO_2 Range (ppm)	Temperature Range (°F)	RH Range (%)
Library (occupied)	474	402–571	64–70	60–73
Main Office (occupied)	505	657–1097	69–73	51–69
Room 108 – Classroom (occupied)	399	492–1288	65–69	64–75
Room 111 – Cooking Lab (unoccupied)	481	395–601	67–69	59–75
Room 203 – Classroom	474	541–1153	66–69	62–83
Room 212 – Classroom (occupied)	475	735–2316	63–68	66–74
Room 213 – Classroom unoccupied	477	440–797	64–69	65–87

Review of Consultant Report

School management hired an environmental consultant to conduct an in-depth IEQ assessment. That evaluation was conducted on March 3-25, 2008. The consultant conducted a visual assessment of all school buildings; evaluated the ventilation systems; checked building pressurization; measured CO_2, CO, temperature, and RH; evaluated total VOCs during the remodeling process; and collected area air samples for mold. They identified problems with the ventilation systems that were addressed before the school reopened in March 2008. They also found fluctuations in RH levels and building pressurization believed to come from leakage around the windows. The consultant found that low levels of total VOCs (1 ppm) were present from the remodeling work and that the levels were decreasing as the work was completed. The mold sampling showed that concentrations were lower in the school buildings when compared to the outdoor concentrations and that the types of mold in both the indoor and outdoor samples were similar.

Employee Interviews

Seven of the 12 employees we interviewed attributed the headache and nausea symptoms that occurred soon after the school was reopened in part to odors from the recent repainting, floor stripping and waxing, and carpet installation. Staff complaints about odors and symptoms to school management reportedly decreased over time after the school was reopened, remodeling was completed, and odors dissipated.

Several employees who reported upper respiratory, sinus, and eye irritation during our September 2007 evaluation were interviewed again in April 2008. Most employees we interviewed who were symptomatic in September 2007 reported that their symptoms improved during the time classes were held at a different middle school, with recurrence of symptoms upon return to this school in March 2008. Most reported these symptoms improved with medical treatment; seven teachers were reassigned to other schools at their request and/or based on physician recommendations. Most staff we interviewed reported concerns about temperature fluctuations in the classrooms, with most stating the rooms were too cold and were uncomfortable for staff and students.

Health Department Investigation

At the request of the school district, staff from the city health department investigated health symptom incidence/school nurse visits among students in the 3 years prior to our 2008 site visit (excluding the approximately 6 months from September 2007 to March 2008 when students were relocated to another school). According to their records review, approximately 50% of visits to the school nurse were a result of injuries, and approximately 50% were due to symptoms such as nausea, stomachache, headache, and dizziness. Only a few respiratory complaints occurred over the 3-year period. Of note, the number of school nurse visits by students was similar in each year of the 3-year period.

2010 Follow-up

In March 2010 we spoke with administrative staff at the middle school to learn whether the classroom windows throughout the buildings had been replaced, as discussed at our April 2008 closing meeting. Additionally, we inquired about reports of health concerns among staff in the year following our second evaluation. We learned that all windows in the facility were replaced in 2008, and the annex building had reopened with no apparent health concerns among staff. Some teachers who previously reported symptoms chose to teach in portable trailers on the middle school campus instead of returning to the regular classrooms.

DISCUSSION

Overall, we found that the mold contamination issues at the school had improved since our 2007 evaluation, although the ventilation units were not reducing RH to the recommended levels. These individual ventilation units were designed to have continuous temperature control but rely on the dehumidification of the cooling system to remove excess humidity from the air. This design is known to have problems maintaining humidity within suggested comfort guidelines in a moderate or hot, humid environment [ASHRAE 2006]. In a humid climate, Lstiburek recommends that the temperature of the outdoor air introduced into the building be lowered to 55°F to dehumidify the air [Lstiburek 1993]. This air is too cold to deliver directly to the classroom without some additional reheat mechanism. The windows were also in disrepair, which likely allowed unconditioned humid air to enter. Since our evaluation, the windows in the school have been replaced. During our evaluation we saw evidence that mold was starting to grow again on some wooden furniture and in unconditioned hallways, likely due to the high RH levels in these areas. Mold spores need water, food, and an acceptable temperature to grow. Because mold spores are always present in the environment, the easiest of these factors to control indoors is the water (i.e., RH).

The ventilation units were clean; two units had water leakage from the drain lines, which was fixed during our visit. The CO_2 levels in Rooms 108, 203, and 212 exceeded the ANSI/ASHRAE recommended guidelines, which can indicate insufficient quantities of outdoor air being introduced into the space. However, adding additional untreated outdoor air can compound the high RH problem. The ventilation units were set to low

Discussion (continued)

temperatures to reduce the RH levels that resulted in comfort issues for the staff. Maintaining comfort parameters (temperature, RH) at recommended levels has been shown to help resolve or improve symptoms among building occupants.

Employee reports of headache and nausea when the school was first reoccupied have resolved with time. These symptoms were likely due to the odors and chemicals from the remodeling activities that were finished just prior to the school reopening. Several of the employees with symptoms in September 2007 had been reassigned to other schools. Individuals who reported upper respiratory, sinus, and eye irritation in September 2007 felt better when they moved to another school and reported that symptoms returned when they moved back to this school. Most of the employees stated that the symptoms responded to medical treatment. The city health department study found no changes in the student health reports during this time period.

Conclusions

We found that the school district had implemented many of the recommendations for the middle school, including regrading soil around the building, repairing pipes in the crawl spaces, and remediating mold. However, work on the ventilation systems was still needed to address cold temperatures, high RH levels, and insufficient outdoor air.

Recommendations

The following recommendations were based on our survey observations, sampling results, and interviews.

1. Consult with a qualified ventilation engineer to provide conditioned 55°F outdoor air (to remove excess RH) to the individual ventilation units. To conserve energy and heat the cold dehumidified outdoor air, air could be recirculated from the classroom through the ventilation system or a heat exchanger. The amount of untreated air entering the classrooms from the hallways should be controlled. Ventilation units in the school should be set to provide 10 CFM of outdoor air per person for classrooms as specified under the Texas Voluntary Indoor Air Quality Guidelines for Government Buildings at http://www.dshs.state.tx.us/iaq/SchoolsGuide.shtm#HVAC_sys. The temperature

and RH should follow current ANSI/ASHRAE comfort guidelines. Because the air in hallways is untreated, the walls between the hallways and classrooms should be treated similarly to exterior walls. This treatment includes limiting the opportunity for air to migrate from the hallways to the classrooms and installing a vapor barrier on the hallway side of the wall.

2. Continue clean-up of the residual mold contamination using appropriate techniques as outlined in the U.S. EPA document "Mold Remediation in Schools and Commercial Buildings" at http://www.epa.gov/mold/pdfs/moldremediation.pdf and the Texas Department of State Health Services mold program at http://www.dshs.state.tx.us/mold/default.shtm.

3. Inform building occupants of the actions taken to address IEQ problems and the rationale for decisions made to address these problems.

4. Start an IEQ management program to address the IEQ issues that have evolved over the past several years and prevent them from recurring. An IEQ manager or administrator with clearly defined responsibilities, authority, and resources should be selected. This individual should have a good understanding of the buildings' structure and function, and should be able to effectively communicate with occupants. Although no comprehensive regulatory standards specific to IEQ have been established, guidelines have been developed by organizations such as ASHRAE, NIOSH, and the U.S. EPA. An employee representative should assist with communication and should be included in the IEQ management program. The NIOSH/U.S. EPA document, "Building Air Quality: A Guide for Building Owners and Facility Managers" may be helpful. A companion NIOSH/U.S. EPA guide, "Building Air Quality Action Plan," can serve as a checklist for developing and assessing an IEQ management program. Additional information specifically for IEQ in schools is available on the U.S EPA website at http://www.epa.gov/iaq/schools/index.html.

5. Encourage employees with potential work-related health concerns to seek evaluation and care from a healthcare provider who is knowledgeable in occupational medicine and IEQ issues.

REFERENCES

ANSI/ASHRAE [2010a]. Ventilation for acceptable indoor air quality. American National Standards Institute/ASHRAE standard 62.1-2010. Atlanta, GA: American National Standards Institute/American Society of Heating, Refrigerating, and Air-Conditioning Engineers, Inc.

ANSI/ASHRAE [2010b]. Thermal environmental conditions for human occupancy. American National Standards Institute/ASHRAE standard 55-2010. Atlanta, GA: American National Standards Institute/American Society for Heating, Refrigerating, and Air-Conditioning Engineers, Inc.

ASHRAE [2006]. Humidity control and design guide for commercial and institutional buildings. Atlanta, GA: American Society for Heating, Refrigerating, and Air-Conditioning Engineers, Inc.

Lstiburek J [1993]. Humidity control in the humid south. Building Science Research Report 9302. [http://www.buildingscience.com/documents/reports/rr-9302-humidity-control-in-the-humid-south] Date accessed: June 2011.

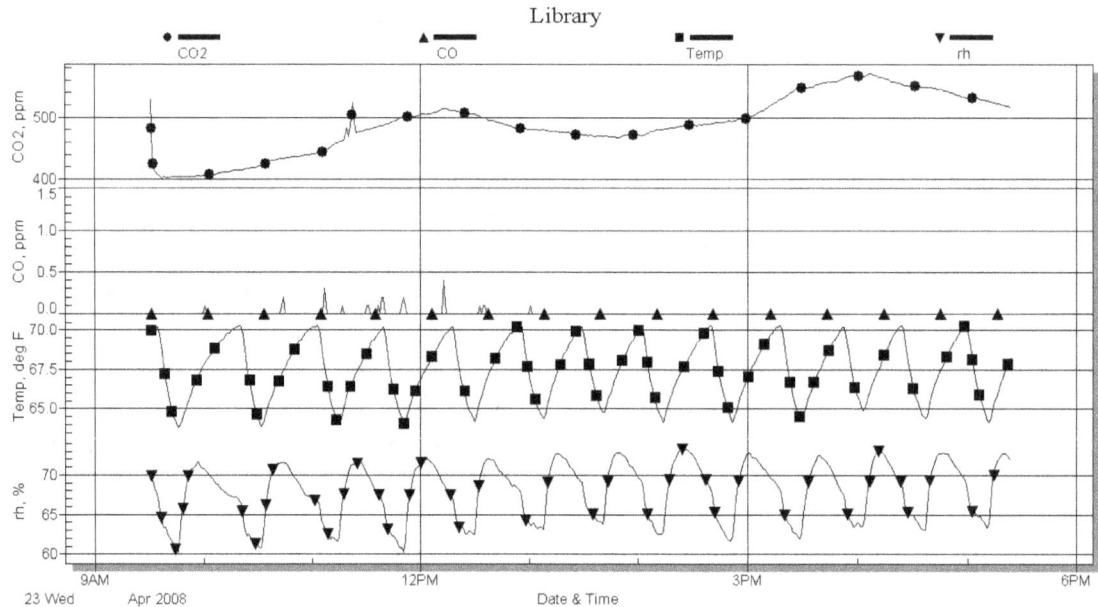

Figure A1. Graph of CO_2, CO, temperature, and RH for the library.

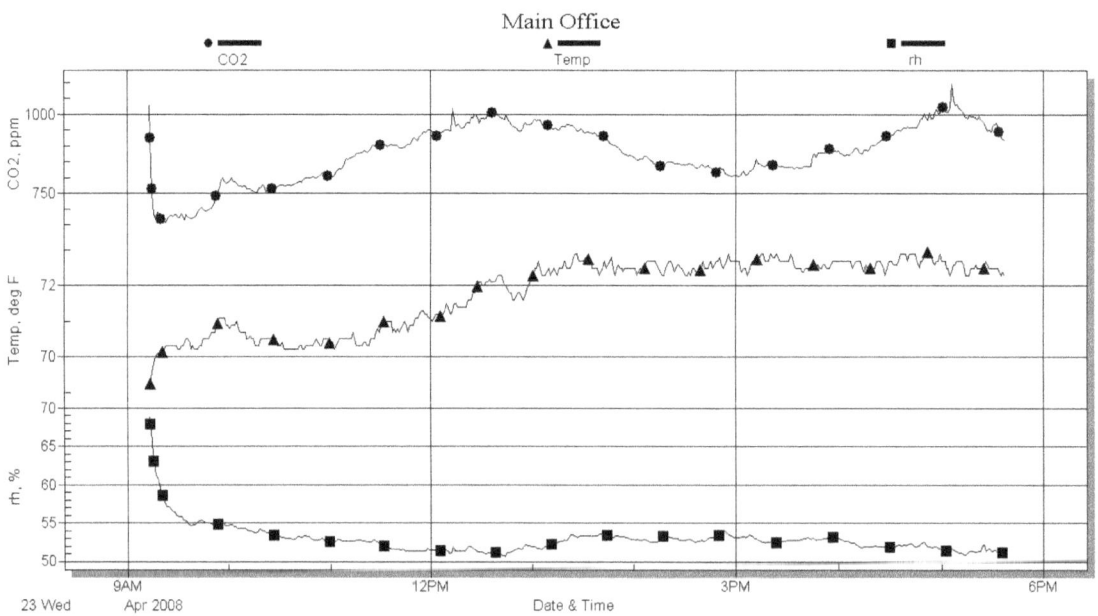

Figure A2. Graph of CO_2, temperature, and RH for the main office.*

*meter had no CO monitoring capability

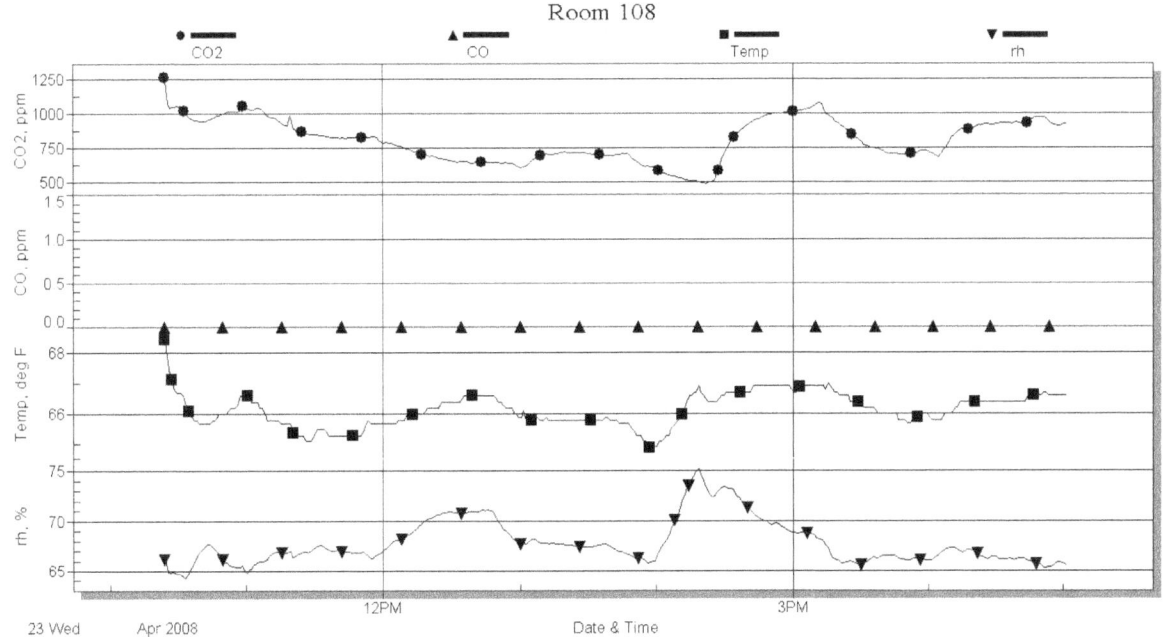

Figure A3. Graph of CO_2, CO, temperature, and RH for Room 108.

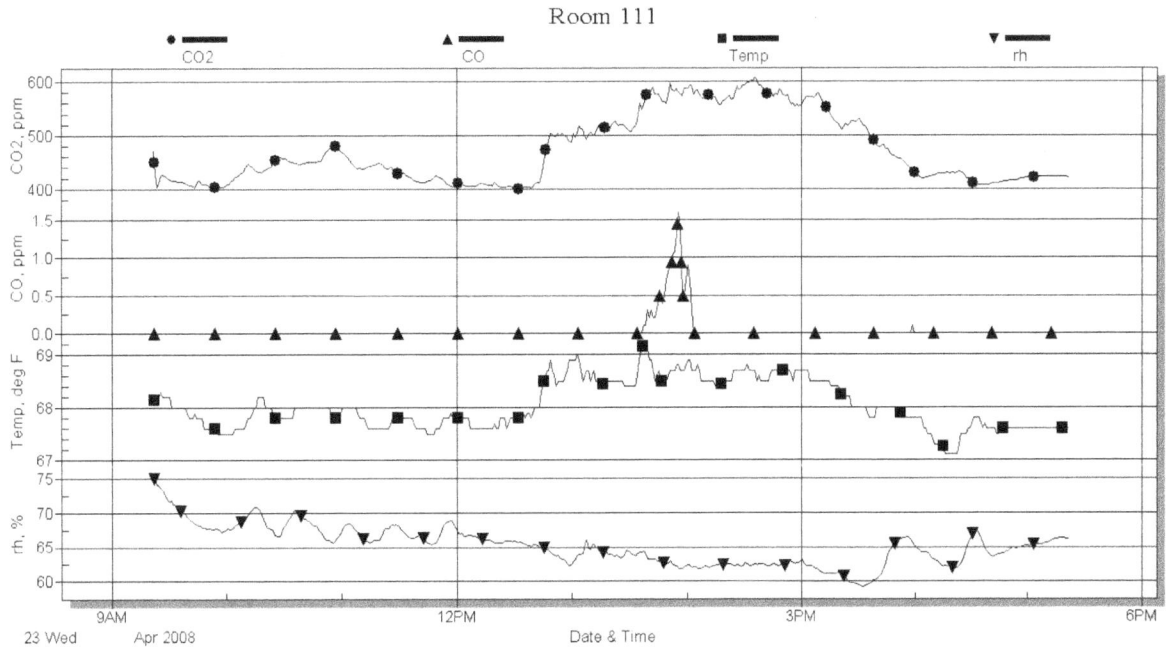

Figure A4. Graph of CO_2, CO, temperature, and RH for Room 111.

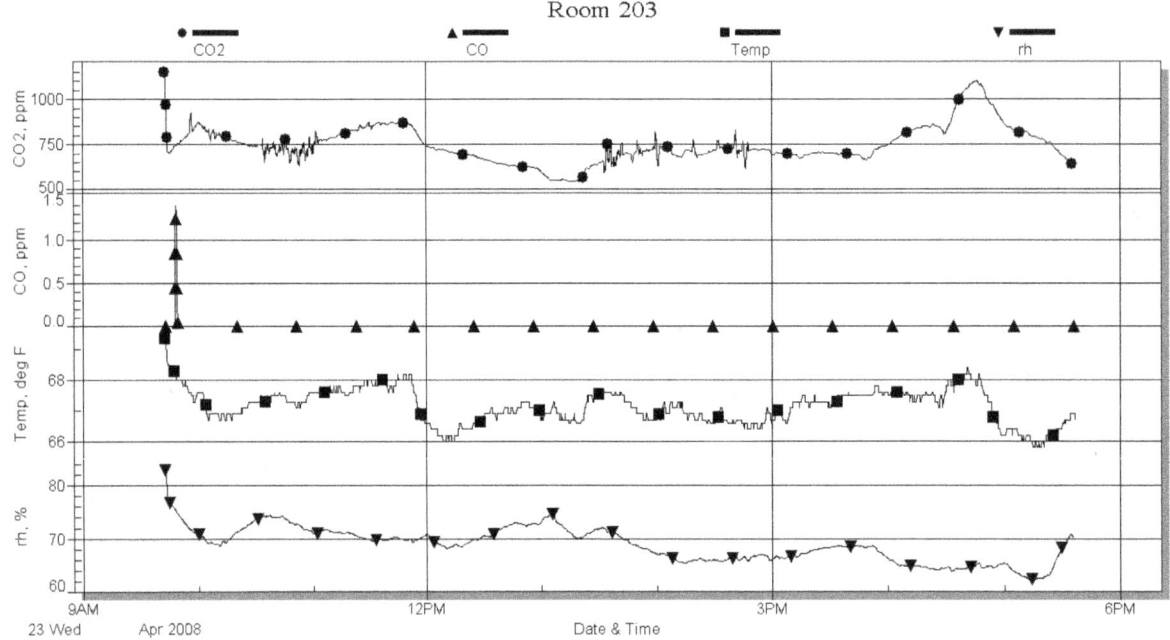

Figure A5. Graph of CO_2, CO, temperature, and RH for Room 203.

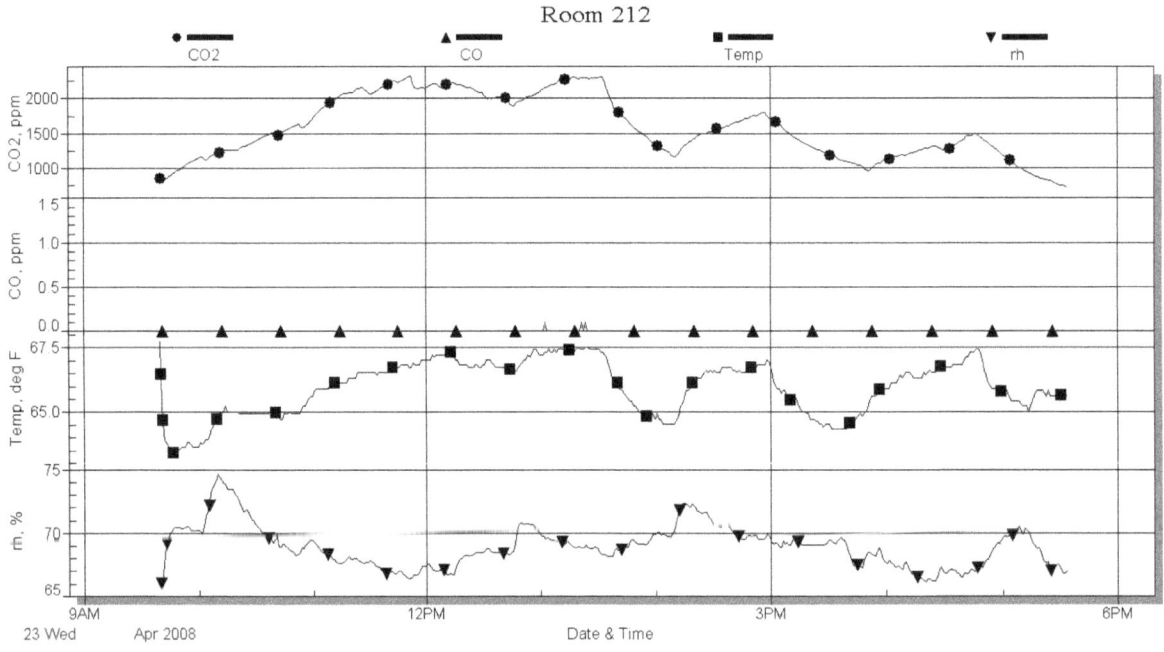

Figure A6. Graph of CO_2, CO, temperature, and RH for Room 212.

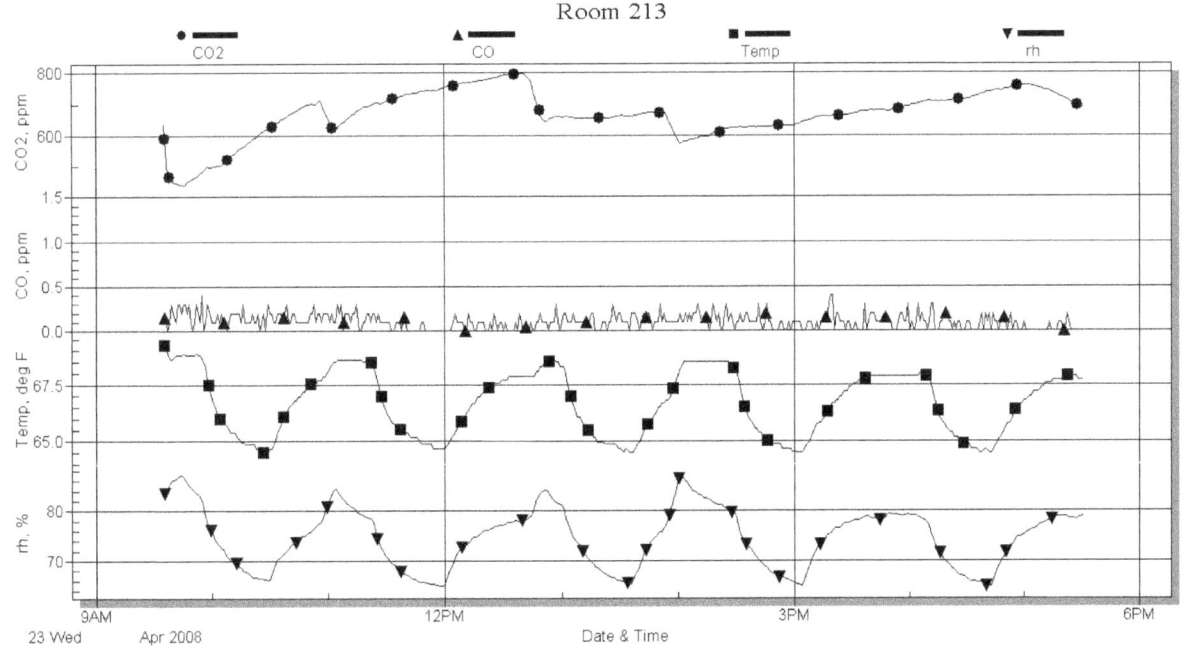

Figure A7. Graph of CO_2, CO, temperature, and RH for Room 213.

Microbial Contamination

Exposure to microbes is not unique to the indoor environment. No environment, indoors or out, is completely free from microbes, even a surgical operating room. Remediation of microbial contamination may improve IEQ conditions even though a specific cause-effect relationship is not determined. NIOSH investigators routinely recommend the remediation of observed microbial contamination and the correction of situations that are favorable for microbial growth and bioaerosol dissemination.

Mold

The types and severity of symptoms related to exposure to mold in the indoor environment depend in part on the extent of the mold present, the extent of the individual's exposure, and the susceptibility of the individual (for example, whether they have pre-existing allergies or asthma). In general, excessive exposure to fungi may produce health problems by several primary mechanisms, including allergy or hypersensitivity, infection, and toxic effects. Additionally, molds produce a variety of VOCs, the most common of which is ethanol, that have been postulated to cause upper airway irritation. However, as discussed above, potential irritant effects of VOCs from exposure to mold in the indoor environment are not well understood. Evidence also shows that exposure to fungal fragments that can contain allergens, toxins, and $(1 \rightarrow 3)$-β-D-glucan may occur [Górney et al. 2002; Brasel et al. 2005; Reponen et al. 2006].

Allergic responses are the most common type of health problem associated with exposure to molds. These health problems may include sneezing; itching of the nose, eyes, mouth, or throat; nasal stuffiness and runny nose; and red, itchy eyes. Repeated or single exposure to mold or mold spores may cause previously nonsensitized individuals to become sensitized. Molds can trigger asthma symptoms (shortness of breath, wheezing, cough) in persons who are allergic to mold. In the 2004 report, "Damp Indoor Spaces and Health," the IOM found sufficient evidence of an association between mold or dampness indoors and nasal and throat symptoms, asthma symptoms in sensitized asthmatics, wheeze, cough, and hypersensitivity pneumonitis in susceptible persons [IOM 2004]. The IOM found limited or suggestive evidence of an association between lower respiratory illness in healthy children and damp indoor spaces. There was inadequate or insufficient evidence to determine whether an association exists between dyspnea, airflow obstruction in healthy persons, mucous membrane irritation, skin symptoms, chronic obstructive pulmonary disease, asthma development, inhalation fevers in nonoccupational settings, fatigue, cancer, reproductive effects, neuropsychiatric effects, lower respiratory illness in healthy adults, gastrointestinal problems, rheumatologic or immune problems, or acute idiopathic pulmonary hemorrhage in infants. No health conditions met the level of evidence for causation. In 2009, WHO published guidelines for protection of public health from mold and other exposures in damp buildings [WHO 2009]. Based on its review of the scientific literature for this report, the WHO concluded that there was sufficient epidemiologic evidence that occupants of damp buildings are at risk of developing upper and lower respiratory tract symptoms (including cough, wheeze, and dyspnea), respiratory infections, asthma, and exacerbation of asthma. The WHO also concluded that limited evidence suggests an association between bronchitis and allergic rhinitis and damp buildings. They noted clinical evidence that exposure to mold and other microbial agents in damp buildings is associated with hypersensitivity pneumonitis.

People with weakened immune systems (immune-compromised or immune-suppressed individuals) may be more vulnerable to infections by molds. For example, Aspergillus fumigatus is a fungal species that has been found almost everywhere on every conceivable type of substrate. It has been known to infect the lungs of immune-compromised individuals who inhale the airborne spores [Wald and Stave 1994; Brandt et al. 2006]. Healthy individuals are usually not vulnerable to infections from airborne mold exposure.

No exposure guidelines for mold in air exist, so it is not possible to distinguish between "safe" and "unsafe" levels of exposure. Nevertheless, the potential for health problems is an important reason to prevent indoor mold growth and to remediate any indoor mold contamination. Moisture intrusion, along with nutrient sources such as building materials or furnishings, allows mold to grow indoors, so it is important to keep the building interior and furnishings dry. NIOSH concurs with the U.S. EPA's recommendations to remedy mold contamination in indoor environments at http://www.epa.gov/iaq/molds/mold_remediation.html [U.S. EPA 2001; Redd SC 2002]. Additional information on health effects and mold remediation can be found in the CDC document "Mold Prevention Strategies and Possible Health Effects in the Aftermath of Hurricanes and Major Floods" at http://www.cdc.gov/mmwr/preview/mmwrhtml/rr5508a1.htm.

No standards specific to the nonindustrial indoor environment exist. Measurement of indoor environmental contaminants has seldom proved helpful in determining the cause of symptoms except where there are unusual sources or a proven relationship between specific exposures and disease. With few exceptions, concentrations of frequently measured chemical substances in the indoor work environment fall well below the recommended OELs published by NIOSH [NIOSH 2005], ACGIH [ACGIH 2011], and AIHA [AIHA 2010], and the mandatory PELs set by OSHA [29 CFR 1910 (general industry)]. ANSI/ASHRAE has published recommended building ventilation and thermal comfort guidelines [ANSI/ASHRAE 2010a; ANSI/ASHRAE 2010b]. The ACGIH and AIHA have also developed a manual of guidelines for approaching investigations of building-related symptoms that might be caused by airborne living organisms or their effluents [ACGIH 1999; AIHA 2008]. Other resources that provide guidance for establishing acceptable IEQ are available through U.S. EPA at http://www.epa.gov/iaq/, especially the U.S. EPA Indoor Air Quality Tools for Schools at http://www.epa.gov/iaq/schools/ and the joint U.S. EPA/NIOSH document, Building Air Quality, A Guide for Building Owners and Facility Managers at http://www.epa.gov/iaq/largebldgs/baqtoc.html.

Heating, Ventilating, and Air-Conditioning

One of the most common deficiencies in the indoor environment is the improper operation and maintenance of ventilation systems and other building components [Rosenstock 1996]. We have found that correcting HVAC problems often reduces reported symptoms. Most studies of ventilation rates and building occupant symptoms have shown that rates below 10 Ls^{-1}/person (which equates to 20 CFM per person) are associated with one or more health symptoms [Seppanen et al 1999]. Moreover, higher ventilation rates, from 10 Ls^{-1}/person up to 20 Ls^{-1}/person, have been associated with further significant decreases in the prevalence of symptoms [Seppanen et al. 1999]. Thus, improved HVAC operation and maintenance, higher ventilation rates, and comfortable temperature and RH can all potentially serve to improve symptoms without ever identifying any specific cause-effect relationships. When conducting an IEQ evaluation, we often measure ventilation and comfort indicators, such as CO_2, temperature, and RH to provide information relative to the functioning and control of HVAC systems.

Carbon Dioxide

CO_2 is a normal constituent of exhaled breath and is not considered a building air pollutant. It can be used as an indicator of whether sufficient quantities of outdoor air are being introduced into an occupied space for acceptable odor control. However, CO_2 is not an effective indicator of ventilation adequacy if the ventilated area is not occupied at its usual occupant density at the time the CO_2 is measured. ANSI/ASHRAE notes in an informative appendix to standard 62.1 that indoor CO_2 concentrations no greater than about 700 ppm above outdoor CO_2 concentrations will satisfy a substantial majority (about 80%) of visitors with regard to odor from sedentary building occupants (body odor) [ANSI/ASHRAE 2010a]. Elevated CO_2 concentrations suggest that other indoor contaminants may also be increased. If CO_2 concentrations are elevated, the amount of outdoor air introduced into the ventilated space may need to be increased. When CO_2 concentrations are used as an indicator to determine outdoor air requirements, ventilation system designs that rely on duct-mounted CO_2 sensors should have some form of ventilation efficiency documentation that relates concentration values observed at the duct location with those observed within the breathing zone of the occupied space.

Temperature and Relative Humidity

Temperature and RH measurements are often collected as part of an IEQ evaluation because these parameters affect the perception of comfort in an indoor environment. The perception of thermal comfort is related to one's metabolic heat production, the transfer of heat to the environment, physiological adjustments, and body temperature [NIOSH 1986]. Heat transfer from the body to the environment is influenced by factors such as temperature, humidity, air movement, personal activities, and clothing. The ANSI/ASHRAE Standard 55-2010: Thermal Environmental Conditions for Human Occupancy, specifies conditions in which 80% or more of the occupants would be expected to find the environment thermally acceptable [ANSI/ASHRAE 2010b]. Assuming slow air movement and 50% RH, the operative temperatures recommended by ANSI/ASHRAE range from 68.5°F to 76°F in the winter, and from 75°F to 80.5°F in the summer. The difference between the two is largely due to seasonal clothing selection. ANSI/ASHRAE also recommends that RH be maintained at or below 65% [ANSI/ASHRAE 2010a]. Excessive humidity can promote the excessive growth of microorganisms and dust mites.

References

ACGIH [1999]. Bioaerosols: assessment and control. Cincinnati, OH: American Conference of Governmental Industrial Hygienists.

ACGIH [2011]. 2010 TLVs® and BEIs®: threshold limit values for chemical substances and physical agents and biological exposure indices. Cincinnati, OH: American Conference of Governmental Industrial Hygienists.

AIHA [2008]. Recognition, evaluation, and control of indoor mold. Prezant B, Weekes DM, Miller JD, eds. Fairfax, VA: American Industrial Hygiene Association.

AIHA [2010]. AIHA 2010 Emergency response planning guidelines (ERPG) & workplace environmental exposure levels (WEEL) handbook. Fairfax, VA: American Industrial Hygiene Association.

ANSI/ASHRAE [2010a]. Ventilation for acceptable indoor air quality. American National Standards Institute/ASHRAE standard 62.1-2010. Atlanta, GA: American National Standards Institute/American Society of Heating, Refrigerating, and Air-Conditioning Engineers, Inc.

ANSI/ASHRAE [2010b]. Thermal environmental conditions for human occupancy. American National Standards Institute/ASHRAE standard 55-2010. Atlanta, GA: American National Standards Institute/ American Society for Heating, Refrigerating, and Air-Conditioning Engineers, Inc.

Brandt M, Brown C, Burkhart J, Burton N, Cox-Ganser J, Damon S, Falk H, Fridkin S, Garbe P, McGeehin M, Morgan J, Page E, Rao C, Redd S, Sinks T, Trout D, Wallingford K, Warnock D, Weissman D [2006]. Mold prevention strategies and possible health effects in the aftermath of hurricanes and major floods. MMWR 55(RR-8):1–27.

Brasel TL, Martin JM, Carriker CG, Wilson SC, Straus DC [2005]. Detection of airborne *Stachybotrys chartarum* macrocyclic trichothecene mycotoxins in the indoor environment. Appl Environ Microbiol 71(11):7376–7388.

CFR. Code of Federal Regulations. Washington, DC: U.S. Government Printing Office, Office of the Federal Register.

Górny RL, Reponen T, Willeke K, Schmechel D, Robine E, Boissier M, Grinshpun SA [2002]. Fungal fragments as indoor air biocontaminants. Appl Environ Microbiol 68(7):3522–3531.

IOM [2004]. Human health effects associated with damp indoor environments. In: Damp indoor spaces and health. Washington, DC: Institute of Medicine, National Academy Press, pp. 183–269.

NIOSH [1986]. Criteria for a recommended standard: occupational exposure to hot environments, revised criteria. Cincinnati, OH: U.S. Department of Health and Human Services, Centers for Disease Control, National Institute for Occupational Safety and Health, DHHS (NIOSH) Publication No. 86–13.

NIOSH [2005]. NIOSH pocket guide to chemical hazards. Cincinnati, OH: U.S. Department of Health and Human Services, Centers for Disease Control and Prevention, National Institute for Occupational Safety and Health, DHHS (NIOSH) Publication No. 2005–149. [http://www.cdc.gov/niosh/npg/]. Date accessed: June 2011.

Redd SC [2002]. State of the science on molds and human health. Statement for the Record Before the Subcommittee on Oversight and Investigations and Housing and Community Opportunity, Committee on Financial Services, United States House of Representatives. Atlanta, GA: U.S. Department of Health and Human Services, Centers for Disease Control and Prevention.

Reponen T, Seo S-C, Iossifova Y, Adhikari A, Grinshpun SA [2006]. New field-compatible method for collection and analysis of β-glucan in fungal fragments. Abstracts of the International Aerosol Conference, St. Paul, Minnesota, p. 955.

Rosenstock L [1996]. NIOSH Testimony to the U.S. Department of Labor on indoor air quality. Applied Occupational and Environmental Hygiene 11(12):1365–1370.

Seppanen OA, Fisk WJ, Mendell MJ [1999]. Association of ventilation rates and CO2 concentrations with health and other responses in commercial and institutional buildings. Indoor Air 9(4):226–252.

U.S. EPA [2001]. Mold remediation in schools and commercial buildings. Washington, DC: United States Environmental Protection Agency, Office of Air and Radiation, Indoor Environments Division. EPA Publication No. 402-K-01-001.

Wald P, Stave G [1994]. Fungi. In: Physical and biological hazards of the workplace. New York: Van Nostrand Reinhold, p. 394.

WHO [2009]. WHO guidelines for indoor air quality: dampness and mould. Geneva, Switzerland: World Health Organization. [http://www.euro.who.int/__data/assets/pdf_file/0017/43325/E92645.pdf]. Date accessed: June 2011.

Acknowledgments and Availability of Report

The Hazard Evaluations and Technical Assistance Branch (HETAB) of the National Institute for Occupational Safety and Health (NIOSH) conducts field investigations of possible health hazards in the workplace. These investigations are conducted under the authority of Section 20(a)(6) of the Occupational Safety and Health Act of 1970, 29 U.S.C. 669(a)(6) which authorizes the Secretary of Health and Human Services, following a written request from any employer or authorized representative of employees, to determine whether any substance normally found in the place of employment has potentially toxic effects in such concentrations as used or found. HETAB also provides, upon request, technical and consultative assistance to federal, state, and local agencies; labor; industry; and other groups or individuals to control occupational health hazards and to prevent related trauma and disease.

The findings and conclusions in this report are those of the authors and do not necessarily represent the views of NIOSH. Mention of any company or product does not constitute endorsement by NIOSH. In addition, citations to websites external to NIOSH do no constitute NIOSH endorsement of the sponsoring organizations or their programs or products. Furthermore, NIOSH is not responsible for the content of these websites. All Web addresses referenced in this document were accessible as of the publication date.

This report was prepared by Nancy Clark Burton and John Gibbins of HETAB, Division of Surveillance, Hazard Evaluations and Field Studies. Ventilation consultation was provided by Kenneth Mead, Division of Applied Research and Technology. Analytical support was provided by Microbiology Specialists Incorporated, Houston, Texas. Health communication assistance was provided by Stefanie Evans. Editorial assistance was provided by Ellen Galloway. Desktop publishing was performed by Greg Hartle.

Copies of this report have been sent to employee and management representatives at the middle school, the state health department, and the Occupational Safety and Health Administration Regional Office. This report is not copyrighted and may be freely reproduced. The report may be viewed and printed at http://www.cdc.gov/niosh/hhe/. Copies may be purchased from the National Technical Information Service (NTIS) at 5825 Port Royal Road, Springfield, Virginia 22161.

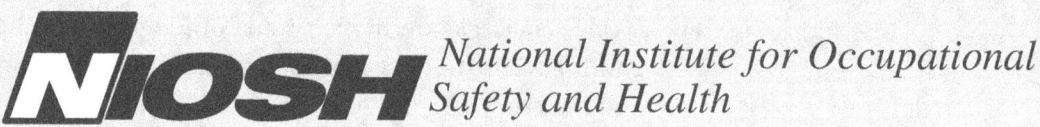

National Institute for Occupational Safety and Health

Delivering on the Nation's promise: Safety and health at work for all people through research and prevention.

To receive NIOSH documents or information about occupational safety and health topics, contact NIOSH at:

1-800-CDC-INFO (1-800-232-4636)

TTY: 1-888-232-6348

E-mail: cdcinfo@cdc.gov

or visit the NIOSH web site at: **www.cdc.gov/niosh.**

For a monthly update on news at NIOSH, subscribe to NIOSH eNews by visiting **www.cdc.gov/niosh/eNews.**

SAFER • HEALTHIER • PEOPLE™

www.ingramcontent.com/pod-product-compliance
Lightning Source LLC
Chambersburg PA
CBHW080941290526
45795CB00007BA/2842